PERIPHERAL NEUROPATHY THRIVING GUIDE

Manage Numbness, Tingling, Pain, And Weakness in The Hands and Feet

Becks Kellyman

Contents

PREFACE

Peripheral neuropathy is a complex and often misunderstood condition that affects millions of people worldwide. It is a condition that causes numbness, tingling, pain, and weakness in the hands and feet, making everyday activities a challenge. Amidst its prevalence, peripheral neuropathy remains a mysterious and often underdiagnosed condition, leaving many patients searching for answers and relief.

This book aims to unfold the mysteries of peripheral neuropathy, providing a comprehensive overview of the condition, its causes, symptoms, proper diagnosis, success stories, and treatment options. Are you a patient thriving with peripheral neuropathy, a caregiver, or a healthcare professional? This book covers the needed knowledge and tools that will help you understand & manage peripheral neuropathy and improve your quality of life.

Chapter One: Introduction Peripheral Neuropathy

Peripheral neuropathy is a condition that affects the nerves outside the brain and spinal cord and can cause a range of symptoms. It's a complex condition affecting millions of people worldwide and significantly impacts their daily lives. So, it's vital to understand what it is, the causes, and how to manage it.

Explaining the term "Peripheral Neuropathy"

"Peripheral" is a Greek word meaning "around." In the context of this book, "peripheral" means outside the "central" nervous system. On the other hand, neuropathy is a combination of two words originating in ancient Greek.

- Neuro: - In Greek, it is called "neuron," which means "nerve."
- Pathy: In Greek, it is known as "pathos," which means "illness" or "disorder."

In Greek, "neuron-pathos" means "nerve" illness or disorder of the "nerve."

Your central nervous system comprises two organs: your brain and spinal cord.

However, the peripheral nervous system covers everything else and includes nerves connected to your brain and spinal cord to supply your face and the rest of your body.

It can sometimes affect internal organs, such as the heart, blood vessels, bladder, or intestines.

The Main Forms of Neuropathies

There are various forms of neuropathy, and I will be taking you through nine (9) different forms for better understanding:

1. **Peripheral Nephropathy:** This affects the nerves in the outer (peripheral) areas of your body, such as your arms, legs, feet, and hands.

2. **Diabetic Nephropathy:** The leading cause of this neuropathy is diabetes. It mainly affects the nerves in the feet and hands. When it involves the nerves controlling your body's automatic functions, it is referred to as autonomic neuropathy.

3. **Autonomic Nephropathy:** This occurs due to damage to the nerves controlling digestion and bladder function, as mentioned above in item 2 (b) of this part.

4. **Focal or Mononeuropathy:** Only one nerve is affected. Examples of this Neuropathy include Bell's palsy and carpal tunnel syndrome (median nerve).

5. **Polyneuropathy:** It affects more than one nerve, and a majority of those with neuropathy have diabetic Neuropathy and HIV polyneuropathy.

6. **Motor Neuropathy**: This condition affects the motor nerves.

7. **Multi-Focal Neuropathy:** It is a progressive muscle worsening condition; men are more common sufferers than women.

8. **Sensory Neuropathy:** Nerves affected in this category are the sensory nerves that control your feelings, such as pain, temperature, or a light touch.

9. Proximal Neuropathy (diabetic poly-radiculopathy.

Stages of Neuropathy

When a test indicates you have neuropathy, knowing the stage of neuropathy is important for your reconstructive plastic surgeon to assess nerve damage and recommend appropriate treatment. Every patient suffering from it passes through these four stages:

Stage One: Numbness and Pain

At this early stage, you will feel that something is "off" with your nerves in your hands and feet. You may feel pain, numbness, or a combination of the two symptoms infrequently.

Stage Two: Constant Pain

At this stage, your pain becomes more noticeable and more difficult to bear. This stage leads to permanent damage.

Stage Three: Intense Pain

Stage three is characterized by worsening pain, usually daily. You may have challenges performing tasks you used to do comfortably without hindrances, such as walking barefoot on the beach.

Stage Four: Numbness/Loss of Sensation (Completely)

If you do not seek treatment for your neuropathy, you will start losing all feelings, and your risk of recurrent wounds and subsequent amputation will increase.

Peripheral neuropathy is the term that covers all nerve conditions affecting a specific subdivision of your nervous system. Various conditions can lead to peripheral neuropathy; what this means is that a lot of symptoms come with this disease. Peripheral neuropathy can affect several parts of your body; this depends on how and why it occurs.

Statistical Presentation of Peripheral Neuropathy

The general prevalence of peripheral neuropathy in adults aged 40 and over was estimated at 28.4% in those with diabetes (4.2 million) and 11.8% in patients without diabetes (14.4 million).

The age, sex, and race-adjusted estimated prevalence rate for peripheral Neuropathy in U.S. adults was 0.5% in those 40 years and over and 1.1% among those greater than 70 years.

About 425 million people worldwide are suffering from this disease, and this number will increase to 628 million people by 2045.

According to a study conducted in Al-Ahas, Saudi Arabia, Type 1 and type 2 diabetes mellitus contribute to a 44.1% global burden of peripheral neuropathy. In the same study, evidence shows that 73.1% of patients with diabetes neuropathy have a low quality of life. At the same time, there is an increase in the risk of low quality of life caused by diabetes neuropathy.

Chapter Two: The Multifaceted Causes

Many factors could lead to peripheral neuropathies, and based on this, it is tough to identify the origin. Any of these factors can lead to Peripheral Nephropathy.

- Injury
- Diabetes
- Systemic disease
- Infections such as Lyme disease, shingles, or AIDS, autoimmune conditions, genetic factors
- Hormonal imbalance
- Toxins
- Medications
- Trauma, Repetitive Stress, and Inflammation
- Vitamin deficiency or poor nutrition
- Kidney or thyroid disease
- Alcoholism
- Environmental factors

Injury

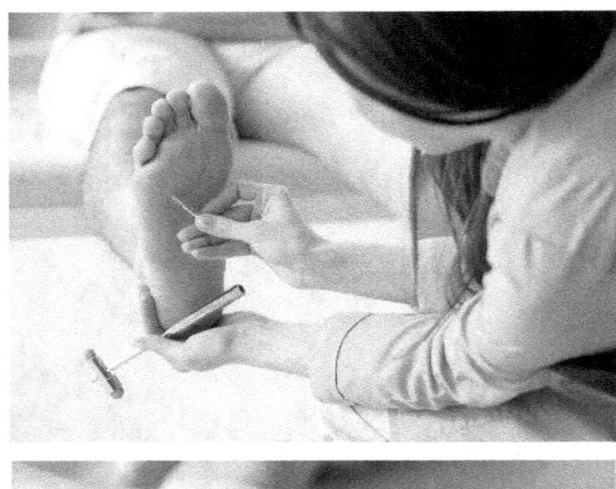

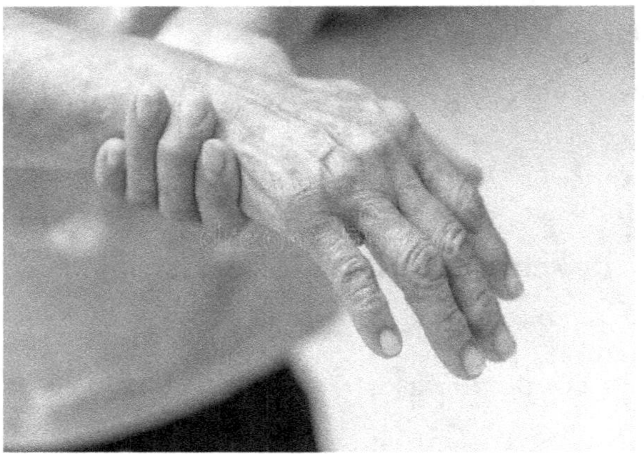

Figure 1

Injury to a peripheral nerve is often related to changes in sensation. Although reduced sensation leading to numbness and tingling is most common, burning, shooting, and sharp electrical-type pains can also occur. Even less severe traumas can cause serious nerve damage, highlighting the importance of seeking medical attention if symptoms persist or worsen over time.

Common Peripheral Nerve Injuries

The following are some of the standard peripheral nerve injuries.

1. Brachial plexus

They split and move down each arm. The main symptom of nerve damage here is sharp pain running from your neck into your shoulder and arm, sometimes with numbness and weakness.

2. Radial nerve injury

It controls your triceps muscles and can extend to your wrists and fingers. If you break your arm, you will have radial nerve injury.

3. Carpal tunnel syndrome

Carpal tunnel syndrome (CTS) is a common health condition that affects the wrist and hand. It occurs when the median nerve, which runs from the forearm into the hand through a narrow passageway in the wrist called the carpal tunnel, becomes compressed or pinched.

4. Ulnar elbow entrapment or bicycler's neuropathy

This nerve branches off the brachial plexus and moves down your arm through your elbow and wrist. Sometimes, it becomes entrapped at the cubital tunnel on the outer side of your elbow. Because the tunnel is tiny, the compression of the nerve will bring pain, weakness, and tingling in your lower arm and hand.

5. Ulnar wrist entrapment

It is similar to carpal tunnel, except different nerves are involved. You are more prone to this type of injury if you bike or play golf, tennis, or baseball.

Diabetes

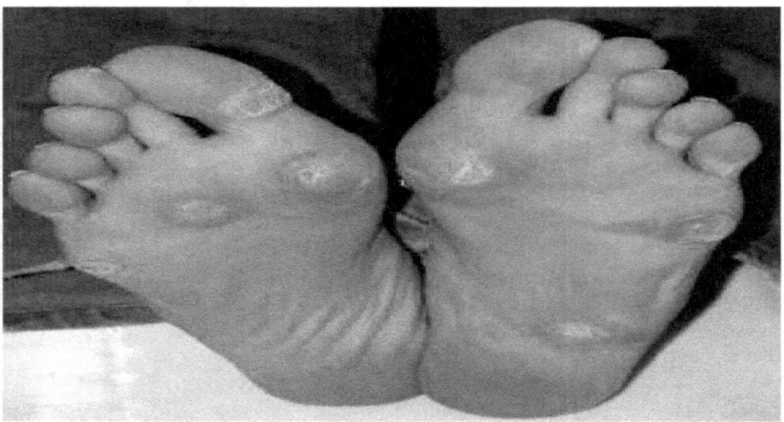

Figure 2

Diabetes is the most common cause of peripheral neuropathy. Diabetic Neuropathy is nerve damage that occurs in people with diabetes.

Systemic Disease

Most peripheral neuropathies result from systemic disease. Peripheral neuropathy resulting from systemic disease refers to any disorder of the peripheral nervous system that is a sequela of a systemic disease process. Systemic disease means disease affecting the entire body rather than a single organ or body part. For example, systemic disorders, such as high blood pressure, or systemic diseases, such as influenza (the flu), affect the entire body.

Infections

Infections may directly damage one or more nerves, usually when the bacteria or virus causes nerve inflammation. You can also end up with nerve damage when the infection triggers an immune response attack against the nerves.

Many different infections can lead to peripheral neuropathy. They are listed here by the name of the bacterium or virus responsible for the infection:

Lyme Disease

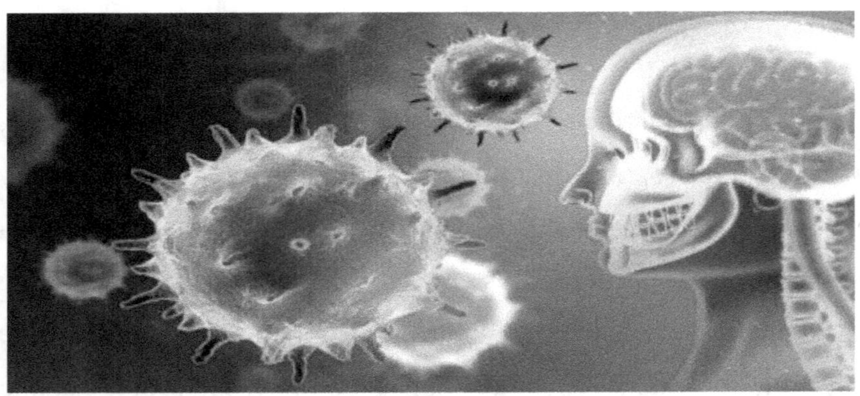

Figure 3

Lyme disease is an infection that happens when an infected tick bites a human. This condition results in joint pain.

The bacteria that cause Lyme disease and its associated infections can affect the central, peripheral, and autonomic nervous systems, leading to a burning sensation in the extremities, lightheadedness with standing, muscle weakness, cognitive impairment, and more.

Shingles (herpes zoster)

Shingles can occur anywhere on your body. Only those previously diagnosed with chickenpox can get shingles. The shingles virus stays dormant in the nerve tissues. If your immune system grows weaker, the virus reactivates and occurs even after the rash disappears.

AIDS

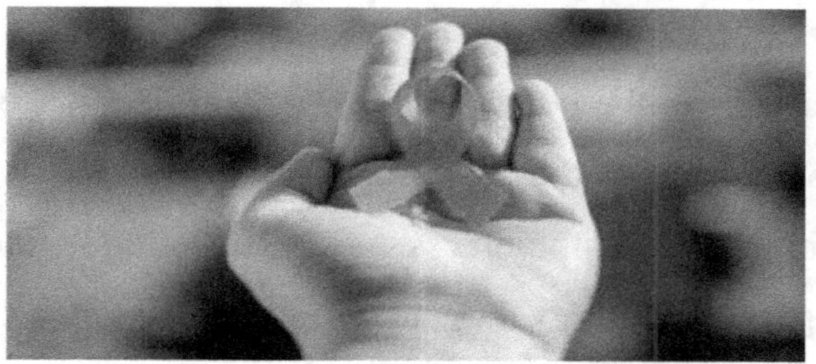

Figure 4

This virus damages your immune system, and HIV interferes with your body's ability to fight infection and disease.

Additionally, 36.7 million people worldwide live with HIV and AIDS, with anywhere from 30% to 60% developing a form of neuropathy.

Damaged nerve fibers can lead to a loss of sensation or weakness in the arms, legs, hands, and feet. The virus infects the nerve cells, leading to cell death. This cell death often damages the long-myelinated fibers, followed by smaller unmyelinated fibers.

HIV-induced peripheral neuropathy, aka "antiretroviral toxic neuropathy," makes up about 2% of those inflicted with peripheral neuropathy in general.

Autoimmune Conditions

The blood cells in the body's immune system help protect against harmful organisms such as bacteria and viruses. These substances contain antigens. The immune system produces antibodies against these antigens that destroy these toxic substances.

The exact cause of autoimmune disorders is unknown.

Areas often affected by autoimmune disorders include:

- Blood vessels
- Connective tissues
- Joints
- Muscles
- Red blood cells

- Skin

Common autoimmune disorders include:

- Addison disease
- Graves' disease
- Rheumatoid arthritis
- Sjögren syndrome
- Systemic Lupus

Sjogren's syndrome, lupus, and rheumatoid arthritis are among the autoimmune diseases that can be associated with peripheral neuropathy.

Genetic factors

There are two hereditary peripheral neuropathies:

- Charcot-Marie-Tooth disease (CMT) is a broad term used to describe a group of inherited neurological disorders characterized by slowly progressive degeneration of the muscles in the foot, lower leg, hand, and forearm, and a mild loss of sensation in the limbs, fingers, and toes.

As the disease progresses, muscle weakness and wasting lead to difficulty walking, running, and balance. Daily activities such as turning doorknobs, fastening buttons, or writing can become arduous if the hands are affected.

- Hereditary neuropathy with liability to pressure palsies (HNPP) is a disorder in which a reasonably mild pressure or trauma to a single nerve results in episodes or periods of numbness and weakness, similar to an arm or leg going to sleep. The most common sites are the wrists, in conjunction with carpal tunnel syndrome, the elbows, and the knees.

These Neuropathies can be categorized by the extent of weakness, sensory involvement, and autonomic involvement; however, overlapping phenotypes make distinguishing inherited disorders from acquired forms challenging.

Hormonal Imbalance

Your hormones are chemical messengers that play a significant role in a series of body functions, from regulating your body temperature to managing complex processes like reproduction and growth. Imbalanced hormones can contribute to weight gain, skin issues, fertility issues, mood changes, irritability, and even neuropathy.

Insulin

Insulin allows glucose to enter your cells, but you have high blood sugar levels when there isn't enough insulin (or your body doesn't use it properly). Over time, unmanaged high blood sugar level damages your nerves, leading to neuropathy.

Testosterone and estrogen

Studies suggest that low testosterone can also contribute to nerve pain. Additionally, low estrogen levels can also increase your risk of developing neuropathy. Unfortunately, both of these hormones tend to decrease with age, so it's even more critical to manage risk factors of neuropathy that you can control. You can manage this situation through weight management, smoking cessation, and regular exercise.

Progesterone

Low progesterone can also impact your nerve health. Low progesterone increases your risk of neuropathy because progesterone supports the healthy formation of the myelin sheath, which is a protective cover surrounding your nerves.

Thyroid hormones

Untreated hypothyroidism can also contribute to peripheral neuropathy. Because hypothyroidism can cause fluid retention, this edema (swelling) can put too much pressure on your nerves. The pressure from swollen tissue can damage your nerves and cause pain.

Toxins/Alcohol/Smoking

More than 200 chemicals exist that are neurotoxic to humans, and drugs or toxins cause 24% of all peripheral neuropathies in the U.S. The segments far away from the nerve body are primarily affected, though certain toxins primarily affect the segments closer in.

What kinds of chemicals cause this neurotoxicity?

Familiar sources of neurotoxin are alcohol, smoking, and illicit drug use. According to the World Health Organization (WHO), 5.1 % of the global cases of disease and injury, including peripheral neuropathy, are related to alcohol and its abuse.

Medications

Did you know that many medications can cause damage to the nerves?

The toxic effect of certain medicines or illicit (street) drugs causes damage to the peripheral nerves.

Many medicines and substances lead to the development of peripheral neuropathy. Examples are listed below.

Heart or blood pressure drugs:

- Amiodarone
- Hydralazine
- Perhexiline

Medications used to fight cancer (chemotherapy drugs):

- Cisplatin
- Docetaxel
- Paclitaxel

Medications used to fight infections:

- Chloroquine
- Dapsone
- Isoniazid (INH), used against tuberculosis
- Thalidomide (used to fight leprosy)

Medications used to treat autoimmune disease:

- Etanercept (Enbrel)
- Infliximab (Remicade)
- Leflunomide (Arava)

Medications used to treat seizures:

- Carbamazepine
- Phenytoin
- Phenobarbital

Anti-alcohol drugs:

- Disulfiram

Drugs to fight HIV/AIDS:

- Didanosine (Videx)
- Stavudine (Zerit)
- Tenofovir and emtricitabine (Truvada)

Trauma, Repetitive Stress, and Inflammation

An injury or swelling can sometimes damage or put pressure on one or more nerves, disrupting their functioning and leading to peripheral neuropathy.

Repetitive stress from work, hobbies, or sports can also put one at risk for peripheral neuropathy. This condition usually affects people between ages 40 and 60, and women are more likely to develop this condition.

Vitamin Deficiencies, Poor Nutrition

When you deprive the nerves of nutrients, they cease functioning correctly. Malnutrition can result from an unbalanced diet (for instance, not enough vitamin B12), diseases, disorders, and drugs that affect the absorption of nutrients into the body.

A deficiency of vitamin B12 can cause cognitive impairment and myelo-neuropathy—damage to the spinal cord and peripheral nerves in the legs—resulting in difficulty walking, weakness, numbness, and poor coordination.

Alcoholism

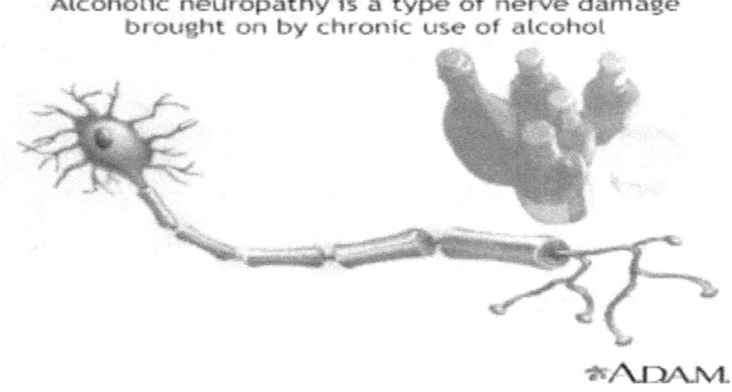

Figure 5

The exact cause of alcoholic neuropathy is unknown.

Environmental Factors

Environmental factors can contribute to peripheral neuropathy in several ways:

1. **Toxic Exposure:** Exposure to harmful substances like heavy metals (lead, mercury, arsenic), pesticides, and industrial chemicals can damage nerves.

2. **Chemical Exposure:** Cleaning agents and solvents can harm nerves.

3. **Radiation:** Radiation therapy can damage nerves, leading to peripheral neuropathy.

4. **Vitamin Deficiencies:** Deficiencies in vitamins like B12, B6, and E can cause peripheral neuropathy.

5. **Hormonal Imbalance:** Hormonal changes can lead to peripheral neuropathy.

6. **Infections:** Certain infections, like Lyme disease, shingles, and HIV, can cause peripheral neuropathy.

7. **Physical Trauma:** Physical injuries, such as car accidents or falls, can damage nerves and lead to peripheral neuropathy.

8. **Repetitive Stress:** Repetitive stress injuries, like carpal tunnel syndrome, can cause peripheral neuropathy.

9. **Exposure to Certain Medications:** Certain medications, such as chemotherapy, can damage nerves.

10. **Environmental Toxins:** Exposure to environmental toxins like mold, pollution, and heavy metals can contribute to peripheral neuropathy.

Chapter Three: Symptoms of Peripheral Neuropathy

The main symptoms of neuropathy can include numbness and tingling in the feet or hands. Loss of balance and coordination. Let us x-ray the different arrays of symptoms associated with peripheral neuropathy below:

Symptoms of peripheral Neuropathy include but are not limited to:

- Extreme sensitivity to touch.
- Sharp, jabbing, throbbing, or burning pain.
- Muscle weakness.
- You will feel as if you are wearing gloves when you are not.
- Slowly experiencing numbness, pricking, or tingling sensation in your hands and feet.
- Experiencing pain while performing activities when ordinarily you are not supposed to.
- Lack of balance
- Falling

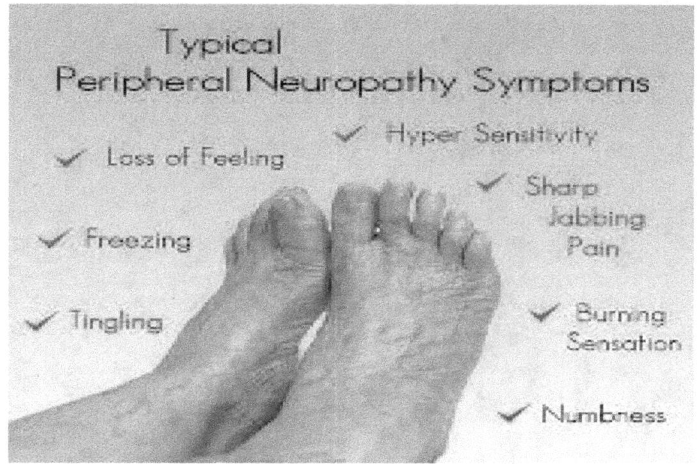

Figure 7

- Drops in blood pressure lead to dizziness or lightheartedness.
- Heat intolerance.
- Bowel, bladder, or digestive problems

Please remember that when peripheral neuropathy affects one nerve, it is mononeuropathy. Suppose it affects two or more nerves in different locations. In that case, it is called multiple mononeuropathy, and if it affects many nerves simultaneously, it is called polyneuropathy. An example of mononeuropathy is carpal tunnel. The majority of persons with peripheral neuropathy have polyneuropathy.

Chapter Four: Diagnosing The Silent Intruder

- These conditions are not life-threatening but can result in damaging symptoms if detected late.
- Early and accurate diagnosis is essential. A delay in diagnosis and precise treatment can cause permanent damage to peripheral nerves.
- Diseases, infections, and accidents can cause damage to the nerve.

So, early and accurate diagnosis is important.

My healthcare provider sent me to a cardio specialist to test my circulation. The results were excellent, and my circulation was okay. My doctor then referred me to another doctor in the same facility because he thought the pains in my leg were a result of neuropathy. On getting there, the doctor agreed that I had diabetic neuropathy.

My neuropathy began five or ten years ago. At first, I thought I stood too long on my feet or overworked myself in the garden and then had leg pains. As time goes, the pain worsened, and that's when I went to my doctor for the first time on this issue. I tried Tylenol at night to reduce the pain, but it didn't help. I started having leg pain continuously, all day and all night.

After my doctor diagnosed me with neuropathy, he prescribed Neurontin, Ultram, and Panalor, which did not help but a little. I noticed the drug made me fall asleep all the time, so I had to reduce the medications. The pain was worse again.

I love dancing a lot, but the pain prevented me from continuing. I must wear high-heeled shoes to work but try to get lower heels. By the end of the work day, my legs are hurting. I don't feel up to anything when I get home. I want to sit down and examine my feet.

I have been very active, and this has slowed me down. I can't go for long walks, shopping (this I love doing), or running around my compound. My diabetes was under control until I lost my job, had no insurance coverage, and had to do without my medication. My sugar level got high, and, of course, the leg pain was severe.

My life has been dramatically affected by this disease because of the pain associated with it. Sometimes, it hurts me so badly that it makes me cry, which only makes me worse. I would be happy if further research and studies would lead to permanent solutions that could remove these pains.

Diagnosis of Peripheral Neuropathy

Apart from a physical examination, such as blood tests, diagnosis usually includes:

- **Your detailed medical history.** Your healthcare professional will look at your complete medical history. The history will cover your symptoms, lifestyle, exposure to toxins, drinking habits, and a family history of nervous system or neurological diseases.

- **Neurological examination.** Your healthcare professional may order the following specific tests:

- **Blood tests.** These can detect low levels of vitamins, diabetes, signs of inflammation, or metabolic issues that could lead to peripheral neuropathy.

- **X-ray examination.** MRI or CT scans can check for pinched nerves, also called compressed nerves, growths, or other problems affecting the blood vessels and bones.

- **Nerve function tests.** Electromyography (EMG) and Nerve conduction studies (NCS) measure and record electrical activity in your muscles to find nerve damage. A thin needle (electrode) is inserted into the muscle to measure electrical activity as you contract the muscle.

- **Other nerve function tests.** These might include an autonomic reflex screen.
- **Nerve biopsy**
- **Skin biopsy.** This procedure removes a small portion of the skin to examine the number of nerve endings.

Nerve Conduction Studies

A nerve conduction study (NCS) – also called a nerve conduction velocity (NCV) test – this test measures how fast an electrical impulse moves across your nerve. NCS can identify nerve damage.

While doing this test, the electrode patches attached to your skin stimulate your nerve. The doctor will place two electrodes on your skin over your nerve, and they function in two capacities: the first stimulates your nerve with light electrical impulses. The second electrode recodes the electrical impulse. Another electrode records the resulting electrical activity. Your healthcare provider will repeat a nerve conduction study for every nerve tested.

A similar test to this is known as electromyography (EMG).

Why conduct NCS?

NCS and an EMG are used to tell the difference between nerve damage and muscle damage.

Conditions or diseases that may require NCS include:

- **Guillain-Barré syndrome.** Your body's immune system attacks your nerves.
- **Carpal tunnel syndrome (CTS).** This syndrome is a usual condition that affects your wrist and hand.
- **Charcot-Marie-Tooth disease.** It is a hereditary motor and sensory neuropathy of the peripheral nervous system characterized by progressive loss of muscle tissue and touch sensation across various body parts.
- **Chronic inflammatory polyneuropathy and neuropathy.** This condition is rare and affects the peripheral nerves. It is a type of neuropathy affecting the nerves outside the brain and spinal cord.

Electromyography (EMG)

Electromyography (EMG) is a diagnostic test to ascertain how healthy a muscle is and the nerve cells that control it (motor neurons). EMG tests can detect a dysfunctional nerve, dysfunctional muscle, or challenges with nerve-to-muscle signal transmission.

An EMG employs tiny electrodes to translate signals into graphs, sounds, or numerical values a healthcare professional can interpret further.

Why an EMG?

Your doctor may request an EMG if you complain of muscle or nerve disorder. Possible symptoms that may require an EMG are as follows:

- Numbness
- Muscle weakness
- Tingling
- Some limb pains
- Muscle pain and cramping

What to note during the study?

During the study, the neurologist will check any ongoing electrical activity when the muscle is resting – an activity not present in healthy muscle tissue – and the activity level as you slightly contract your muscle.

Blood Tests to Identify Underlying Causes

The under-listed blood tests are carried out to identify the underlying causes of peripheral neuropathy:

- Complete blood count (CBC)
- Comprehensive metabolic panel
- Thyroid function test
- Tests for vitamin-12levels
- HbA1C
- Tests for metals and minerals
- Tests for infections
- Tests for inflammation and autoimmunity
- Tests for blood and bone marrow cancers and potential cancers

Collaboration Between Health Care Professionals and Peripheral Neuropathic Patients to Pinpoint the Exact Type and Cause of Peripheral Neuropathy.

Sub-classifications can be made by separating peripheral neuropathies as axonal, demyelinating, or mixed, which is essential for treatment and management.

Etiology of Peripheral Neuropathy

Peripheral neuropathies can come from a variety of origins, including metabolic, systemic, and toxic causes. Below is the etiology you will consider:

- Diabetes mellitus
- Hypothyroidism
- Chronic alcoholism
- Guillain-Barre syndrome
- Chemotherapy agents
- Inflammatory conditions (e.g. vasculitis)
- Trauma/injury
- Multiple myeloma
- Hereditary conditions (e.g., familial amyloidosis, Charcot-Marie-Tooth disease)
- Toxins (heavy metals, chemicals)
- Infections (e.g., Epstein-Barr virus, Lyme disease, Epstein-Barr virus, hepatitis C, Shingles, Leprosy)
- Medications (antibiotics, cardiovascular medications)
- Monoclonal gammopathy of undetermined significance (MGUS)
- Tumors (secondary to compression or associated paraneoplastic syndrome)

In some instances, an actual cause may be unknown.

Complications of Peripheral Neuropathies

The complications of peripheral neuropathy include pain, altered sensation, muscle atrophy, and weakness. Diabetic peripheral neuropathy is infamous for complications, including foot ulcers, which can lead to dangerous digits and limbs, sometimes progressive to amputation.

Healthcare Professionals to Consult

List of consultants and referrals for peripheral neuropathy patients.

- Physical therapist
- Endocrinologist
- Neurologist
- Hematologist/oncology (for those with neuropathy related to cancer
- Infectious disease specialist
- Rheumatologist
- Occupational therapist
- Psychiatry & addiction medicine (for those with alcohol-induced peripheral neuropathy)
- Chronic pain physician
- Surgeon (for neuropathy secondary to compression).

Educating the Patient

Peripheral neuropathic patients require education on the signs and symptoms of this condition. Patients should be informed that they have an increased risk of injury due to loss of sensation; they should be conscious of any new cuts or damage to their skin as wound healing can be delayed, and the risk for infection rises.

I recommend you always wear socks with closed-toed shoes to reduce the risk of infection. It would help if you were cautious when exposing yourself to hot or cold environments to avoid burns and frostbite. If you have diabetes, you should receive counseling on managing your diabetes properly. If you are a patient with alcohol-induced peripheral neuropathy, ensure you get adequate information on cessation.

Enhancing Healthcare Team Collaboration

A lot of diseases can lead to peripheral neuropathies, which routinely need an inter-professional team approach to diagnosis and treatment. This team should include specialists, physicians, specialty-trained nurses, and, when necessary, pharmacists, all working in collaboration to achieve optimal patient care and outcomes. Thus, it is essential to equip yourself as a professional with a prompt diagnosis of the underlying condition followed by the initiation of appropriate treatment(s) to reverse, slow, or stop the progression of the disease.

Identifying patients most at risk for neuropathies and implementing a preventative approach to their care can undoubtedly improve outcomes, as in the case of diabetic neuropathy. As primary care providers and nurse practitioners are often the first to work with these patients, they must be familiar with the full range of etiologies that play a part in the development of peripheral neuropathies, including testing and referrals to the right specialists.

Chapter Five: Empowerment Through Understanding

Peripheral neuropathy is usually linked with specific psychological and emotional feelings: fear as a result of painful sensation and suspicion of danger associated with various activities may lead to irritability and social withdrawal.

Stress can push the body to release certain hormones, such as cortisol or adrenaline. These hormones can cause damage to the nerves and result in inflammation, leading to cell damage. As this situation continues, it can lead to neuropathy and disorders related to nerves. Apart from physical impact, stress can also greatly affect your mental health.

Emotional Ways of Coping with Peripheral Neuropathy

It is never an easy task living with neuropathy. If the condition has lasted for a long time, you may feel angry, sad, and hopeless as a result of persistent pain. You will feel the urge to withdraw from close friends and families or stop doing your daily routines.

Here are five ways to take charge of those emotions and cultivate better thoughts. Your mind is responsible for behavior — and can be used to make positive changes in one's life.

1. Practice self-care.

Surround yourself with friends, family, and people who give you support. Participate more in activities you love, such as bringing you joy.

2. Managing your stress level.

The technique that works very well when you are at home or trying to sleep is progressive muscle relaxation. The result is that it relieves anxiety.

3. Talk about how you are feeling.

4. Control those feelings you can.

Reducing the amount of inflammatory foods you eat can help you feel better physically.

If your nerve pain affects your sleep, consider small changes you can make.

5. Seek physical relief from pain.

You don't have to live with nerve pain. There is a treatment known as Intraneural Facilitation (INF). With INF, pressure is applied to different parts to increase blood flow and lower pain.

Empathic Stories of Neuropathic Patients

Anna's story

My name is Anna, and I have a chronic condition called peripheral neuropathy. I have lived with this condition for over ten years, and I am okay with it now!

How it all started

My journey started in my early 40s when I experienced numbness in my right calf. It was something that I was not concerned about; I did not notice any hurt or change in my movement, so I moved on with my life. Later, I observed that I kept tripping over things that were not there. My foot did not lift like it used to. I started asking myself what was happening to me! Oh well, I still went about my daily activities.

I immediately knew I had injured it, but my guy told me to walk it off!

This surgery ignited the lion that was sleeping in my body. Within a matter of days, my toes started hurting. I thought my cast was too tight. I blamed the pain on the surgery. My therapists were a little confused.

Patrick's story

In 1985, at the age of 45, I was diagnosed with a small-fiber length-dependent sensory peripheral neuropathy. When the diagnosis was first made 40 years ago, I was told the disorder would be progressive, but I did not know what that might mean.

I could not discern temperature or pinpricks in my feet, and when I touched things, my hands and feet would tingle. It was uncomfortable to keep my shoes on for long periods. Friends would notice that I would take my shoes off whenever I sat down, and they would give me a hard time. But life went on.

With the passage of years, the neuropathy progressed, as was predicted. The sensory loss became more profound, and my feet and ankles felt numb all the time. I thought I was wearing socks, even when I wasn't. Then, autonomic imbalances emerged and took their toll. It is hard to keep my balance, and with the loss of proprioception, I would never trust myself to walk any distance in the dark.

And then, for several years now, there is pain.

Lancinating pain. A thousand cuts.

Could I still tell the difference between the pain and the fear it generated?

How to Seek Support from Healthcare Professionals?

Seeking support from healthcare professionals is crucial in managing peripheral neuropathy. Here's a step-by-step guide to help you get the needed support:

1. **Primary Care Physician:** Begin with consultation with your primary care physician, who can evaluate your overall health and refer you to a specialist.
2. **Pain Management Specialist:** If you are experiencing chronic pain, consider consulting a pain management specialist for guidance on pain relief options.
3. **Physical Therapist:** A physical therapist can help you maintain muscle strength and mobility through exercises and physical therapy.
4. **Neurologist:** A neurologist specializes in treating nerve disorders and can diagnose and manage peripheral neuropathy.

5. **Mental Health Professionals:** Living with peripheral neuropathy can be challenging, so consider seeking support from a mental health professional for stress and anxiety management.
6. **Podiatrist:** If you have foot or ankle symptoms, consult a podiatrist for proper foot care and prevention of complications.
7. **Occupational Therapist:** An occupational therapist can assist with daily activities and recommend adaptive devices to improve functionality.

Before Your Appointment

1. Keep a symptom journal to track your symptoms and any changes you may be experiencing.
2. Write down your medical history, including previous diagnoses and medications.
3. Prepare a list of questions to ask your healthcare provider.

During Your Appointment

1. Feel free to share your concerns with your healthcare provider.
2. Ask questions and seek clarification on any unclear information.
3. Discuss treatment options and develop a personalized plan.

Seeking support from support groups

Seeking support from a support group for peripheral neuropathy can be incredibly beneficial. Here's how to seek support:

1. **Find a Local Support Group:** Search online or contact organizations like the Peripheral Neuropathy Foundation or the Neuropathy Association to find local support groups.
2. **Online Support Groups:** Join online forums, social media groups, or online support communities, like the Peripheral Neuropathy Support Group or the Neuropathy Support Group.
3. **Attending Meetings:** Attending support group meetings to connect with others who understand your journey.
4. **Share Your Story:** Share your experiences, symptoms, and challenges with the group.
5. **Listen to Others:** Listen to others' stories, advice, and experiences.
6. **Ask Questions:** Ask questions and seek guidance from others who have faced similar challenges.
7. **Offer Support:** Offer support, encouragement, and validation to others in the group.
8. **Participate in Activities:** Group activities, like educational events, webinars, or fundraising campaigns.

9. **Build Relationships:** Build relationships with group members and stay connected between meetings.
10. **Be Open-Minded:** Be open-minded to others' new ideas, treatments, and coping strategies.

Support groups offer a safe space to share your journey, receive emotional support, and connect with others who understand your experiences.

The purpose of the group is to:

- Provide opportunities for patients to help patients;
- Educate patients with basic information on neuropathy;
- Assist patients in discovering practical solutions for patient symptoms;
- Involve patients in community outreach by dispensing educational information.
- Create an atmosphere of hope and encouragement;
- Empower patients with neuropathy knowledge;
- Help patients find a neuromuscular neurologist in their area.

Seeking Support from Loved Ones

Seeking support from your loved ones is essential when living with peripheral neuropathy. Here is how to seek the support you need:

1. **Open Communication:** Share your feelings, symptoms, and challenges with loved ones.

2. **Specific Requests:** Ask for specific help, like accompanying you to appointments or assisting with daily tasks.

3. **Educate Them:** Help them understand peripheral neuropathy, its effects, and how they can support you.

4. **Emotional Support:** Lean on loved ones for emotional support, encouragement, and validation.

5. **Join a Support Group:** Consider joining a support group to connect with others who understand your journey.

6. **Be Open to Help:** Accept help when offered, and don't be afraid to ask for it when necessary.

7. **Show Appreciation:** Express gratitude for their support and care.

8. **Involve Them in Care:** Encourage loved ones to participate in your care, like attending appointments or helping with medication reminders.

9. **Support Their Support:** Recognize the emotional toll of caregiving and offer support and encouragement to your loved ones.

10. **Celebrate Milestones:** Celebrate small achievements and milestones together, like managing a flare-up or completing a physical therapy session.

By seeking support and building a strong support network, you can:

1. Feel more empowered and in control.
2. Better manage symptoms and flares.
3. Improve your mental and emotional well-being.
4. Enhance your overall quality of life.

Continue pushing forward, and remember you are not alone in this journey!

Skills for Coping with Peripheral Neuropathy

Some of these suggestions may help you or your loved one cope:

1. **Set Priorities:** Decide which tasks your loved one must do on a given day, which should be basic, such as bathing, grooming, and eating.
2. **Accept and Acknowledge:** Encourage your loved one to accept and acknowledge the negative aspects of their illness, but then progress forward to embrace positivity and find daily solutions that curb the pain.
3. **Visit Often:** Those who have severe pain, especially in hospice, often can't get their minds off it. It surrounds them every day.

4. **Get Moving:** To the extent your loved one can make sure you get daily exercise, even if it is walking up and down the hall or even the driveway.

5. **Have Them Talk to A Counselor or Therapist:** Therapy is often a part of hospice. Encourage your loved one to speak to a therapist about their pain as they approach the end of life.

Chapter Six: Crafting A Comprehensive Management Plan

On a general note, peripheral neuropathy can be managed in diverse ways, but I have highlighted the steps below to help you manage it.

Prevention is better: Minimize your neuropathy risk; you must maintain your blood sugar levels at equilibrium.

Early diagnosis and treatment. It can help prevent more serious problems. For example, treating a foot infection can prevent the need for serious medical interventions, such as amputation.

Pay attention to other health challenges: Health conditions, such as unidentified elevated blood pressure, can worsen neuropathy. Collaborate with your healthcare provider to provide a better management plan for these conditions.

Ensure weight reduction: Be active for 120 minutes each week – you can do this in shorter sessions. You can replace sugary drinks with water. Eat foods with less sugar and fat content. Discuss your weight loss plan with your family, friends, loved ones, and healthcare providers.

Modification of Lifestyle

Lifestyle modification is the ability to change long-term habits for the better, basically food and other physical activities and sustaining the new habit for a long period.

Lifestyle modification can be used to treat a series of health conditions, including diabetes, obesity, and peripheral neuropathy.

Diet

Eat a good meal. A diet containing fruits, potatoes, avocados, quinoa, and leafy vegetables within an acceptable limit can form part of your plan to manage your weight, lowering the risk of developing peripheral neuropathy.

These five plant-based foods are great for your health and help lessen your pains.

Fruits: Eat at least one fruit a day; it helps repair damaged nerves. Fruits such as cherries, oranges, red grapes, berries, watermelon, peaches, and others are highly rich in antioxidants, which are helpful in the reduction of inflammation and nerve damage.

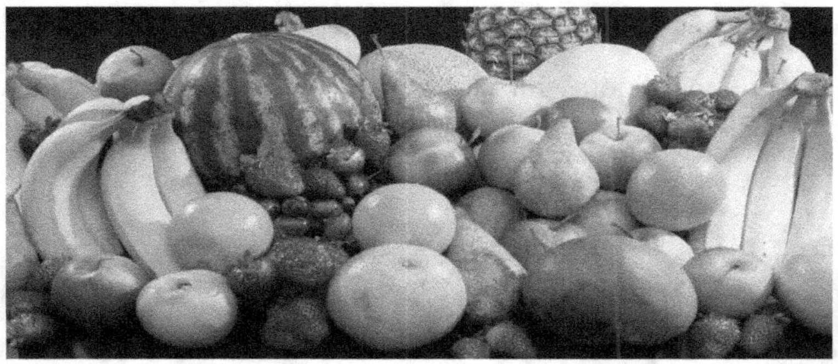

Figure 9

Potato: Sweet potato is rich in vitamins A and C, which contain antioxidants for cell protection. Animal research has proven that eating sweet potato extract has greatly reduced nerve and brain tissue inflammation.

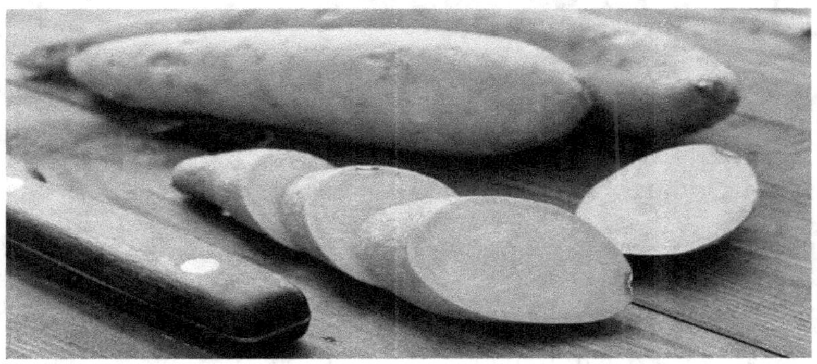

Figure 10

Avocado: This exceptional fruit is very rich in healthy fats. It has a healthy amount of potassium, which enhances active nerve function. Avocados also help your body absorb more antioxidants.

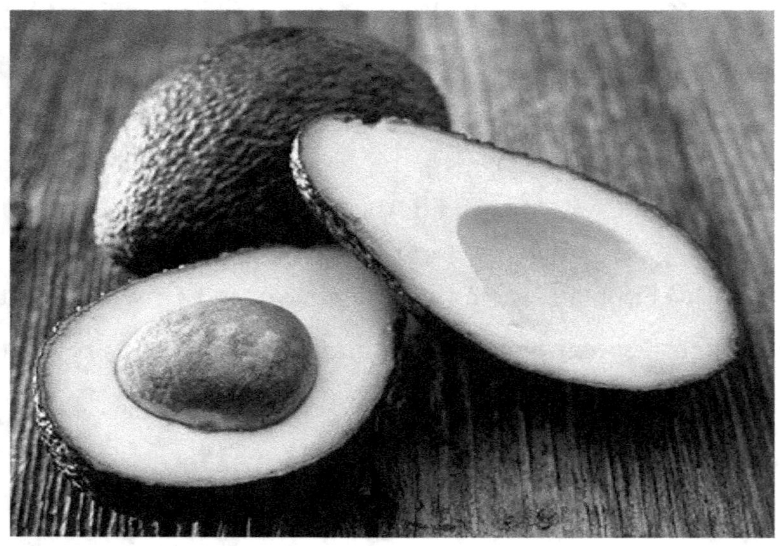

Figure 11

Quinoa: Quinoa is commonly known as a grain; it is a flowering plant with eatable seeds. Like avocado, it has a healthy dose of potassium, which helps active processing of information through nerves. It is very rich in manganese, phosphorous, magnesium, and folate.

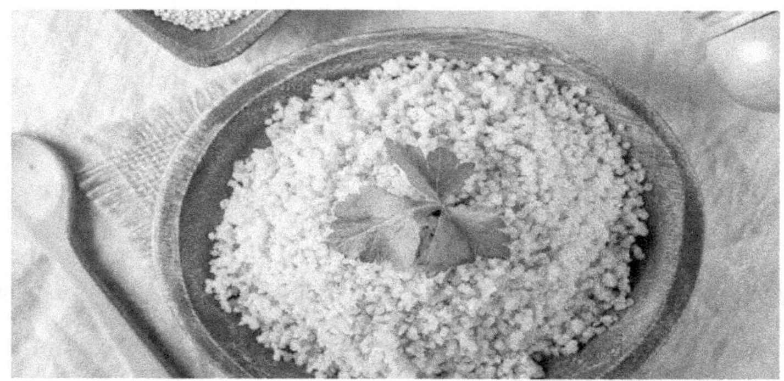

Figure 12

Leafy vegetables: Vegetables such as spinach, broccoli, and asparagus all contain vitamin B. This nutrient is necessary for nerve recreation and proper functioning.

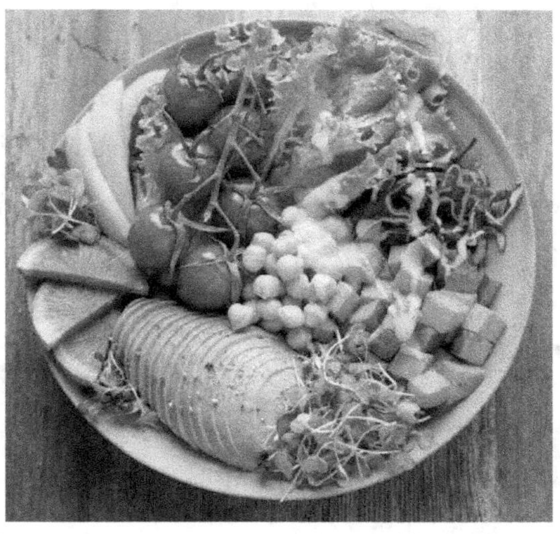

Figure 13

Exercise

Three major categories of exercise are recommended for people with peripheral neuropathy: aerobic, balance, and stretching.

Aerobic exercise: This is a type of exercise that strengthens your heart and lungs. The aerobic exercises that help relieve pains from peripheral neuropathy are cycling, rope jumping, cardio kickboxing, dance, swimming, and running.

Balance exercise: Walking, heel-to-toe, heel raises, and single-leg standing are known as balance exercises, and they help improve balance as they strengthen the legs and feet.

Stretching: These are various types of stretching exercises that you can engage in: PNF stretching, quadriceps stretching, ballistic stretching, hamstring stretching, cat-cow, shoulder stretching, isometric stretching, dynamic stretching, butterfly stretching, and cobra stretching.

Medications for Pain Relief and Symptom Management

Various medication options are available for peripheral neuropathy, which includes antidepressants, anticonvulsants, non-opioid pain relievers, nonsteroidal anti-inflammatory drugs, adjuvants analgesics, and little opioids. Some of these drugs come with side effects, while others have moderate to no side effects. Please note that you must consult your healthcare provider before taking the under-listed medications for pain and symptom management.

Antidepressants. The following are the most effective antidepressants for peripheral neuropathy: tricyclic antidepressants (TCAs) and serotonin-noradrenaline reuptake inhibitors (SNRIs).

Anticonvulsants. These neuropathy medications act on specific ion channels that traffic calcium ions. And they include gabapentin (Neurontin) and pregabalin (Lyrica).

Little opioids. The medications under this category are Tramadol (Ultram), tapentadol, morphine, and oxycodone.

Non-opioid pain relievers. The drugs under this category include aspirin, acetaminophen, ibuprofen, ketoprofen, and naproxen.

Nonsteroidal anti-inflammatory drugs. They are diclofenac and indomethacin. Others have been mentioned under non-opioid.

Adjuvants analgesics. The drugs in this range are cox-2 inhibitors (celecoxib and rofecoxib), muscle relaxants (baclofen, carisoprodol, cyclobenzaprine, diazepam, orphenadine, metaxalone, and tizanidine.

Physical Therapy

Physical therapists play a vital role in helping individuals improve and maintain functions that peripheral neuropathy may limit.

Physical Therapy aims to relieve pain, help you move better, or strengthen weakened muscles. Another vital goal is to show you what you can do yourself to promote your health.

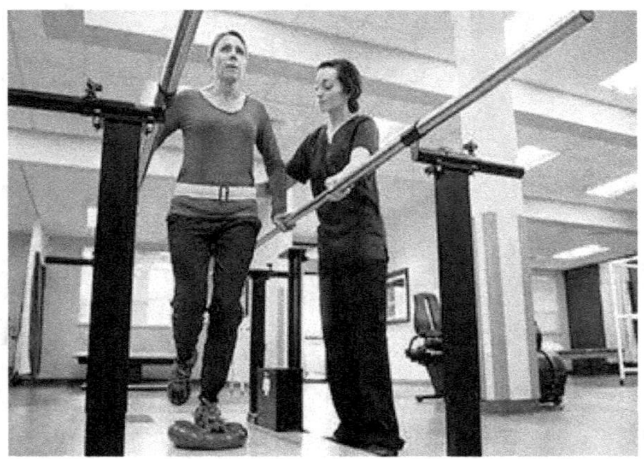

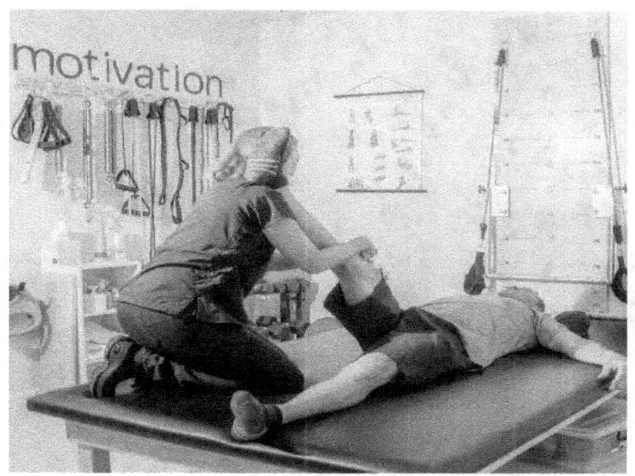

Figure 14

Because peripheral neuropathy's cause, type, and symptoms can vary, the approach to care will also vary. Your physical therapist may recommend the following care:

Moderate-intensity exercise.

Moderate-intensity exercise are those activities that keep you moving strenuous enough to burn down two to seven times as much energy each minute as you do while exercising generally.

The following are considered moderate-intensity exercises for PN.

- Easy jogging.

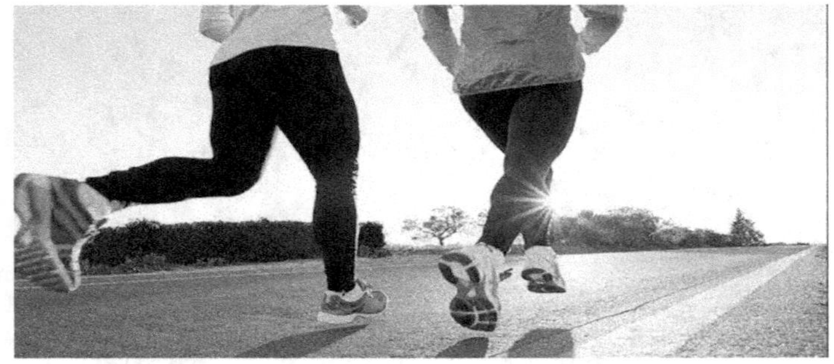

Figure 15

- Water aerobics.

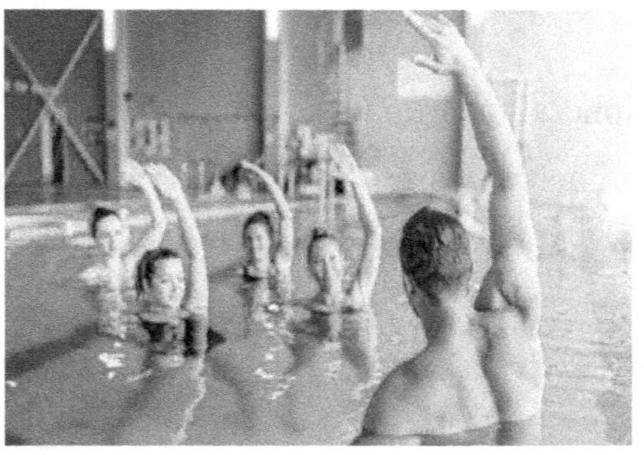

Figure 16

- Using an elliptical trainer.

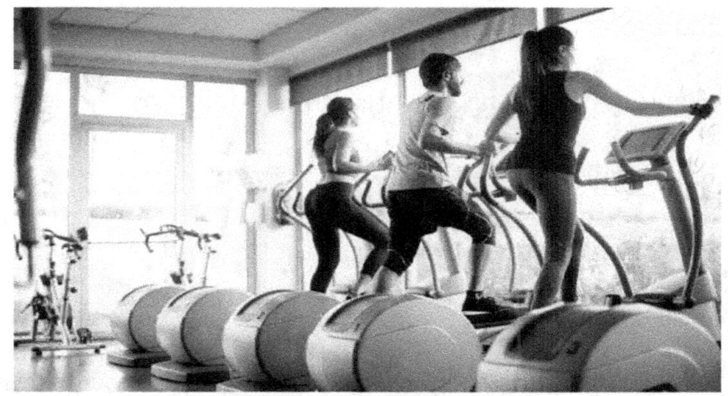

Figure 17

- Swimming leisurely.

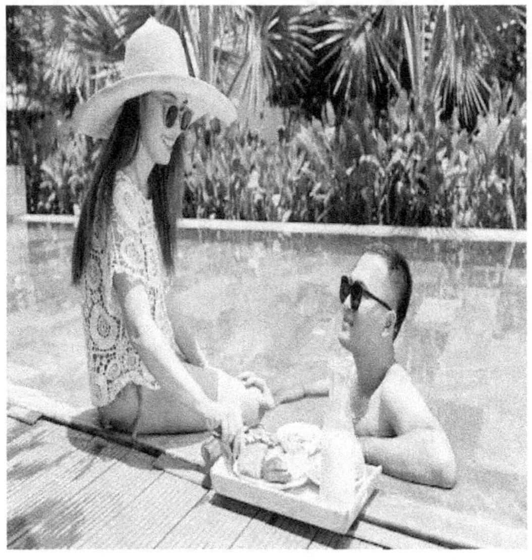

Figure 18

- Ballroom dancing and line dancing.

- Walking or jogging on a treadmill.

- Brisk walking

- Bicycling under 15 miles each hour, on level ground or with few hills.

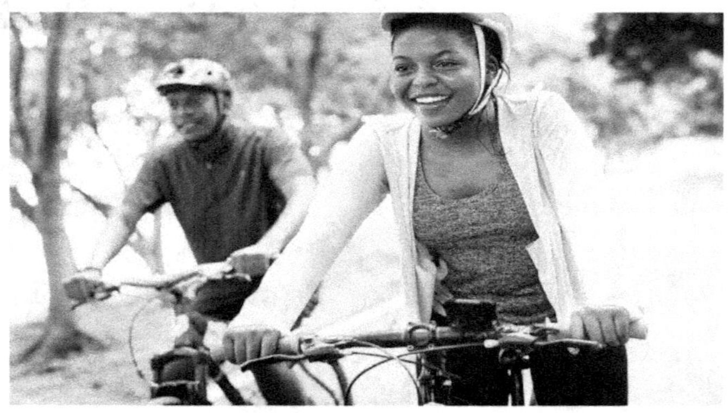

Figure 19

- Riding a bike.

- Hiking.

- Pushing a lawn mower.

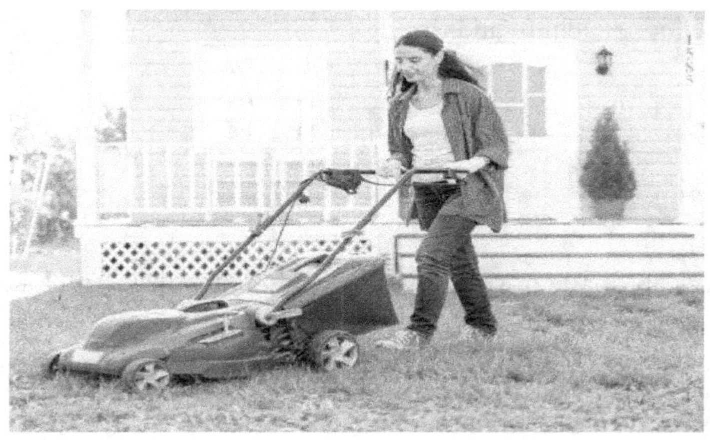

Figure 20

Balance and coordination activities.

These are activities or exercises performed on one foot while you remain standing for some time at home or when you are out and about. It can also be referred to as an action involving standing up from a seated position without using your hands or trying to walk in line, heel-to-toe, for a short distance.

Single-limb stance. Stand straight behind a chair and hold on to the back of it for support and balance.

- Make a heel-to-toe walk

- March on the spot.

- Clock reaching and timing.

- Perform heel-to-toe raises.

Bracing.

Braces are made of soft, durable fabric but can also include plastic, metal, and Velcro straps.

Below are some abdominal bracing exercises you can try at home:

- Pelvic floor exercises.

- Alternate arm and leg raise exercises.

- Heel slide exercise.

- Side plank.

- Forward plank – modify this exercise to reduce the load on your pelvic floor by engaging in these exercises while kneeling instead of being on your toes.

Education.

Patient education includes providing information about your conditions and treatment options and identifying and modifying any factors or activities causing your pain. Instructions on home pain and swelling management, as well as a home exercise program, will help maintain gains in motion and strength.

Occupational Physical Therapy

Occupational Therapy is an allied health profession that deals with the everyday use of therapeutic activities or occupations to treat the physical, mental, developmental, and emotional ailments that impact a patient's ability to perform their daily roles.

Occupational physical Therapy aims to help you live your life more independently. This form of treatment is more useful if you have limited use of your hands and legs as a result of peripheral neuropathy.

Five common occupational physical therapy activities you can engage in:

Adapting to Your Daily Routines. Your therapist may encourage you to:

Using a one-handed rocker knife while cooking is important because activities such as cutting with knives can be harmful, even if you don't have sensory reactions.

You should go for Velcro shoes or elastic laces to handle other issues arising from difficulty tying shoes using your hands.

Home modifications. Modifying your home involves actions you take to ensure smooth movement in and around your home.

If you notice a limited sensation in your feet, ensure you add adequate lighting to your walkways. It will help minimize falls while you are walking.

Management of pain. Your therapists can recommend pain management methods in the following ways – acupuncture, Reiki, cupping yoga, and mindfulness.

A new way of living. It would help if you talked with your therapist about better ways of living with your condition.

It would help if you protect your hands using gloves during activities such as cooking or gardening. Wearing gloves helps protect your skin and also reduces your risk of having an infection.

Physical examination. Your therapist can provide you with a method of examining yourself daily to find out if there are cuts or scrapes on your hands and feet. This is to rule out potential infections as a result of wounds of which you were not aware at all.

You can do this by placing a mirror below your bed and sliding it out each night to inspect visually the bottom of your feet easily.

Alternative Therapies

The alternative medicine open for peripheral neuropathy patients is acupuncture, chiropractic techniques, and energy-based modalities, which include Reiki.

Acupuncture

This procedure is a form of alternative medicine whereby fine needles are placed inside the skin at a particular point along what is known to be lines of energy, used in treating different health conditions, including pains from peripheral neuropathy.

Acupuncture Techniques

You want to ask how many acupuncture points we have in our body; the answer is simple. Chinese traditional medicine has identified 2,000 acupuncture points. This treatment will be targeted at various points, and the treatment depends on the particular symptom in question. These points are located along invisible paths in the body called "meridians."

12 major acupuncture meridians in your body

For easy viewing, the picture below shows the 12 major acupuncture meridians in our body as lines. The acupoints are the points along the lines that are related to each meridian.

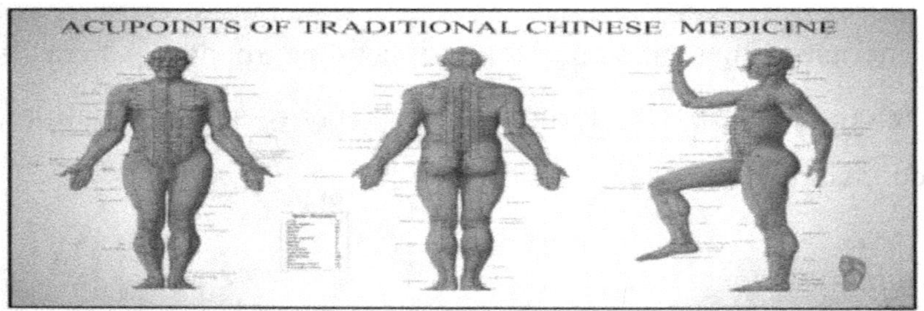

Figure 21

Here are 12 major meridians in our body named based on the organ they are connected to:

- Heart

- Liver

- Lung

- Kidney

- Bladder

- Small intestine

- Large intestine

- Stomach

- Spleen

- Pericardium

- Gallbladder

- Triple burner

Steps in selecting acupuncture points to relieve pain

There are three steps in selecting acupuncture points, and they are as follows:

Step 1: figure out the affected meridian

As soon as the actual place where the pain is coming from is identified, your acupuncturist will then locate the affected meridian(s). for instance, Bladder meridian is associated with upper back and shoulder pains.

Step 2: identify the meridians that will stand in for the affected meridian.

Five other meridians will balance every affected meridian—for example, Heart – kidney, gallbladder, small intestine, bladder, spleen.

Step 3: Select the acupuncture points

Since we have now identified some of the balancing meridians, it is time to select acupoints along them.

Where to needle on leg	Pains in areas of head % trunk	Where to needle on arm
Hip joint,	Neck, jaw, base of skull,	Shoulder
Knee	Waist, L2	Elbow
Ankle	Genitals, bladder, sacrum	Wrist
Toe	Testicles, anus	Finger
Lower leg,	Lower abs, back	Forearm
Top of hip	Top of head	Top of shoulder
Foot	Genitals, coccyx, lower sacrum,	Hand
Upper leg	Chest, mid-upper back,	Upper arm

Table 1

Chiropractic

Chiropractic is a form of treatment whereby a chiropractor, who is a practitioner in chiropractic, makes his hands to help relieve conditions affecting the bones, joints, and muscles.

Chiropractic Techniques:

All chiropractors have preferred techniques and may adopt specific techniques according to what they know about the patient and their associated condition. There are five chiropractic techniques I shall share with you.

Gon stead techniques: In this technique, a chiropractor adjusts the lower back or pelvis. The patient is expected to lie on their side while performing this technique. With this position, the chiropractor realigns your joints, which may cause stiffness, pain, or hinder a person's general movement.

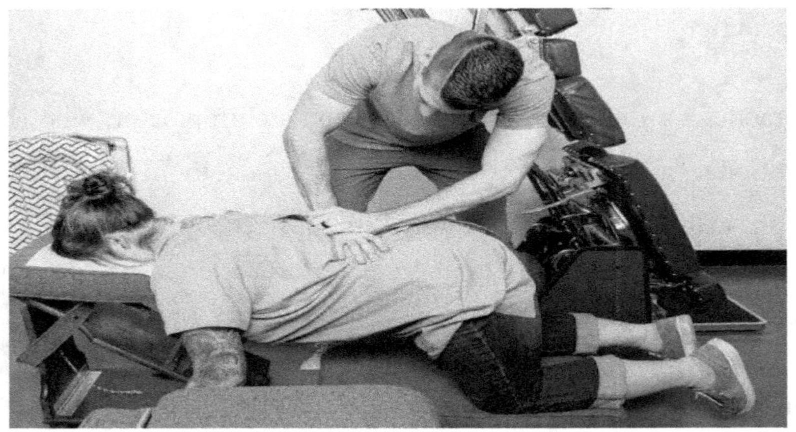

Figure 22

Extremity manipulation: As the name implies, this technique applies joint manipulation outside of the spine. For instance, extremity manipulation may involve physically manipulating the elbow, wrist, knee, shoulder, hip, and ankle joints.

This technique can be used for several conditions but is common for patients with carpal tunnel or posture-related conditions.

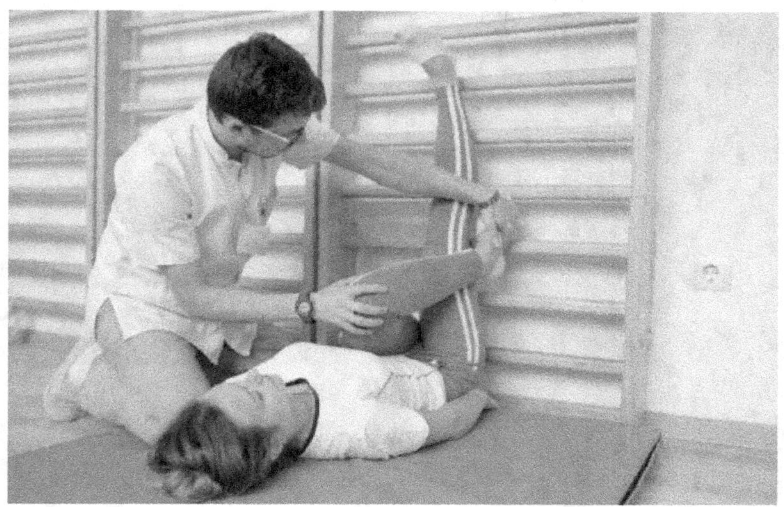

Figure 23

Flexion distraction: The chiropractor makes use of a special table, which allows for the manipulation of the patient's spine position. Together with the table motion, the chiropractor uses manual techniques to remove pressure from the disc.

Activator method: The activator technique is important for the alleviation of back and neck pain in the region outside the spine. In this technique, the chiropractor uses a specific activator-adjusting instrument.

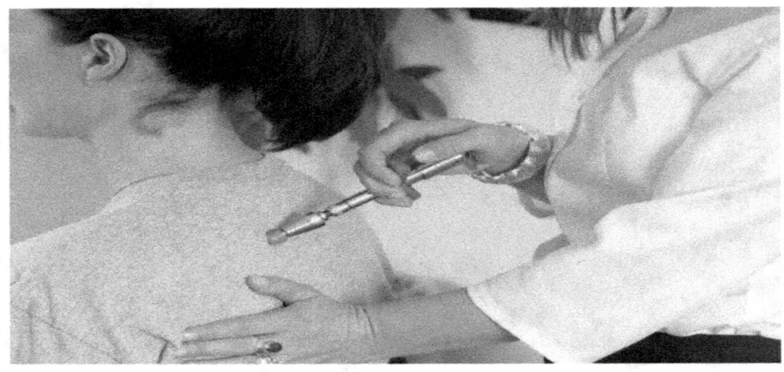

Figure 24

Spinal manipulation: This technique aims to restore and improve joint function in the spinal column.

Spinal manipulation applies a gentle thrusting motion together with stretching to activate the joints and improve their movement.

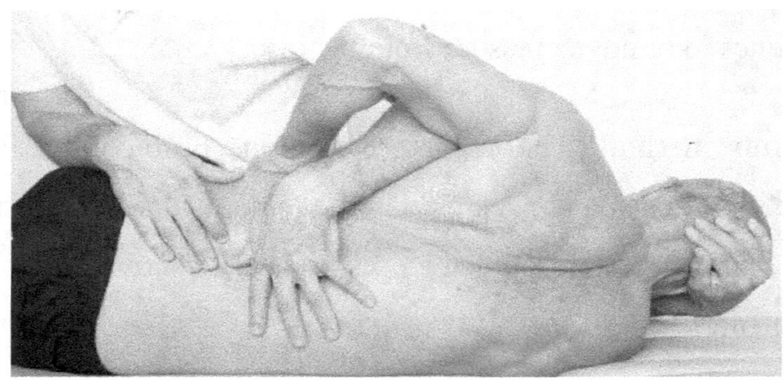

Figure 25

Reiki

Reiki is a type of healing energy. According to Practitioners, the energy can remain stationary in the body where physical injury or pain has occurred. As time goes on, this stagnation of energy can lead to illness.

Energy therapy is aimed at helping the flow of energy and removing blocks in a way that is similar to that of acupuncture. Practitioners of Reikists believe that the flow of energy around the body can promote relaxation, relieve pain, enhance healing, and reduce other symptoms of the disease.

Reiki procedures:

Reiki is administered in a private, peaceful setting. However, the treatment can be done anywhere. In this procedure, the patient is expected to sit in a comfortable chair or lie on a table, covered fully with clothes.

The hands of the practitioner are then placed lightly over or on particular sections of the patient's head, limbs, and torso. Their hands will be maintained in these positions for at least 4-12 minutes.

For those with specific injuries, for example, burns, the practitioner will hold their hands just after the wound.

When the practitioner notices that energy or heat flow in their hands has stopped, they will remove their hands from that particular spot and position it over a different location in their body.

Below are Reiki techniques that cannot be covered in this book due to limited space.

- Clearing
- Infusing
- Centering
- Smoothing and raking the aura
- Beaming
- Extracting harmful energies

Yoga

Yoga is basically a spiritual exercise tied to optimal partial science, mainly focused on harmonizing the body and mind. It is an art and science which promotes healthy living.

Poses are the cornerstone of yoga. Poses are very good to learn as you build a regular practice in yoga.

Ten yoga poses for your practice

Child's Pose

This pose gradually stretches your lower back, hips, thighs, knees, and ankles and relaxes your spine, shoulders, and neck.

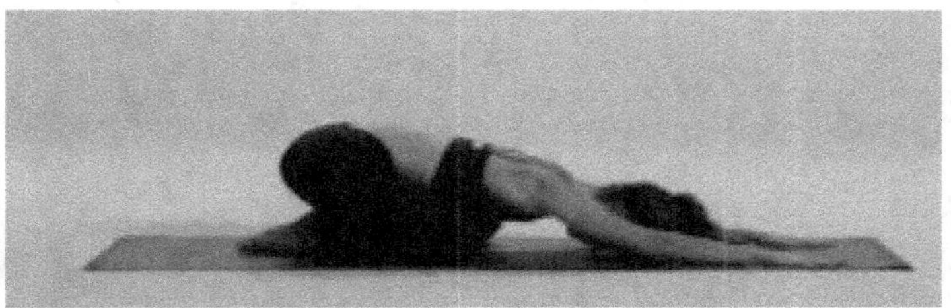

Figure 26

Dog Facing-Downward Pose

Dog facing downward adds strength to the arms, shoulders, and back while stretching the hamstrings, calves, and arches of your feet.

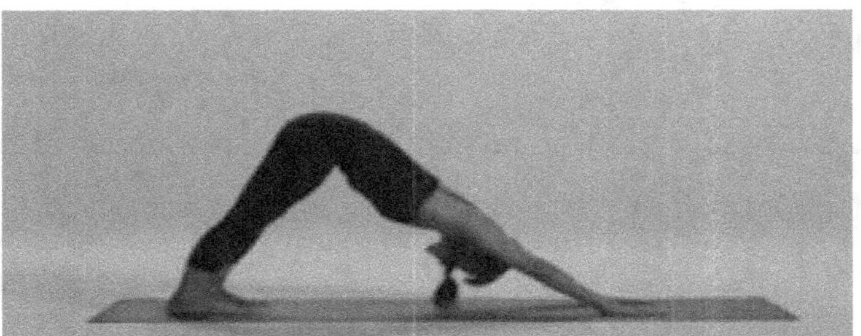

Figure 27

Plank Pose

With the plank pose, you can easily build strength in the arms, legs, core, and shoulders.

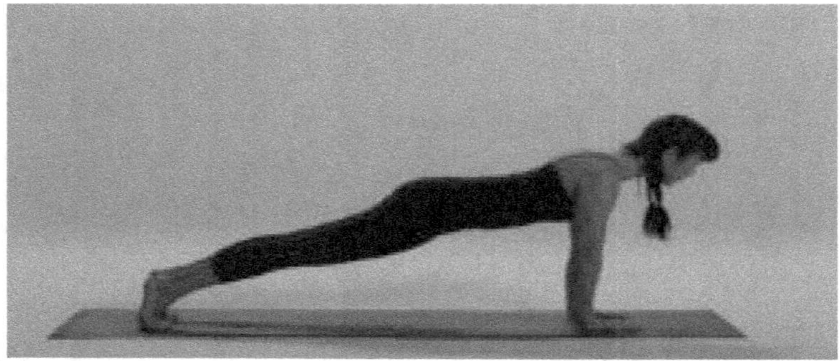

Figure 28

Four-Limbed Staff Pose

This pose is next to the plank pose, which is a push-up variation and a common yoga sequence mostly known as the sun salutation.

To do this pose, press your palms evenly into the floor and lift your shoulders away from the floor as you hold this pose.

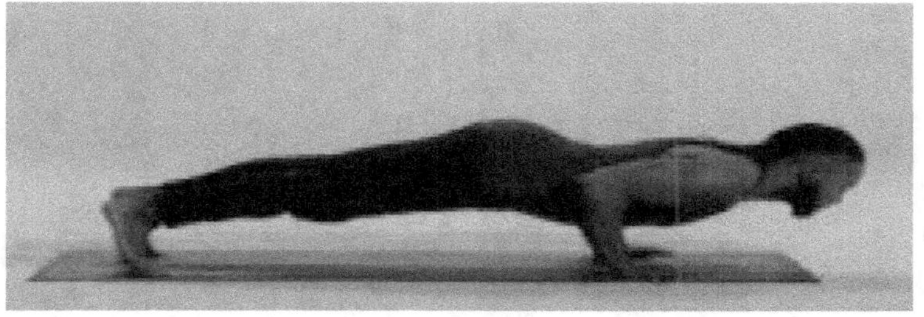

Figure 29

Cobra Pose

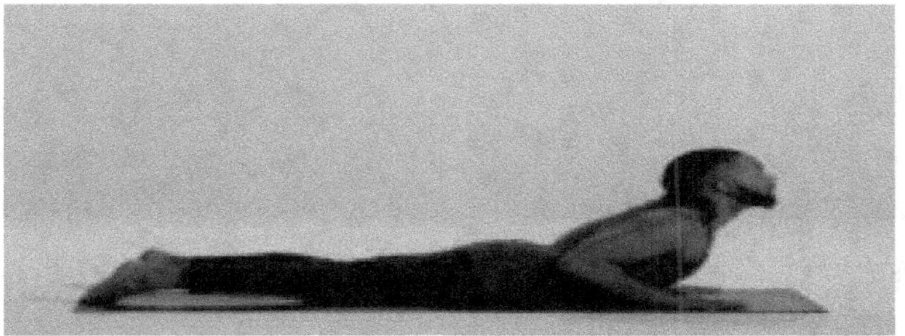

Figure 30

Tree Pose

Apart from helping to improve your balance, it also adds strength to your ankles, calves, cores, thighs, and spine.

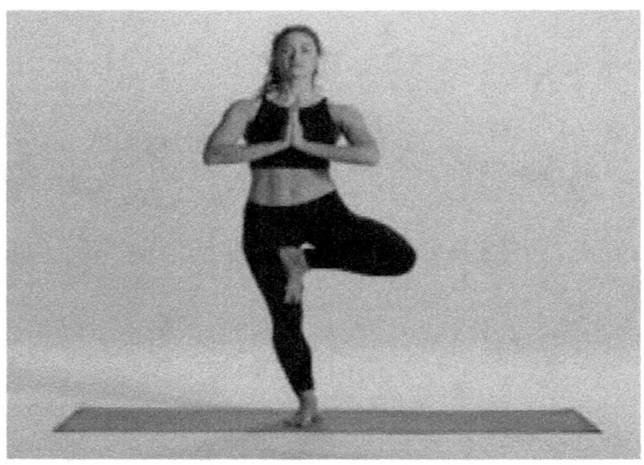

Figure 31

Triangle Pose

Triangle helps build strength in the legs and stretches the hips, spine, chest, shoulders, groins, hamstrings, and calves. It also helps improve movement in the hips and neck.

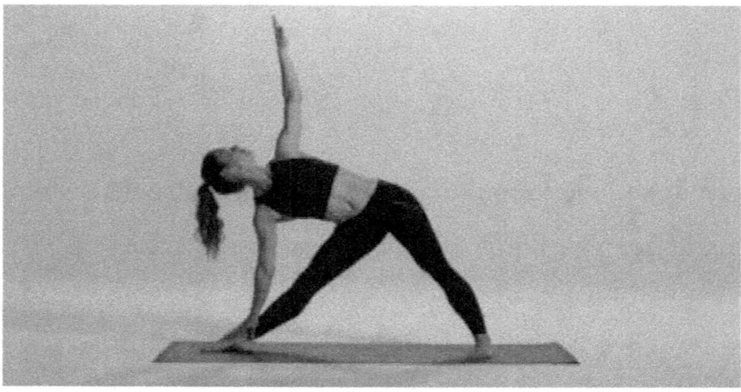

Figure 32

Seated Half-Spinal Twist Pose

This twisting pose increases the flexibility in your back while stretching the shoulders, hips, and chest. It also relieves tension in the middle of your back.

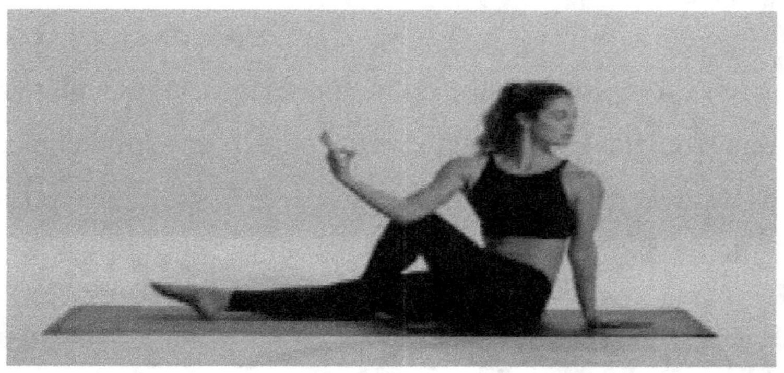

Figure 33

Bridge Pose

This type of back-bending pose stretches the muscles of the back, chest, and neck.

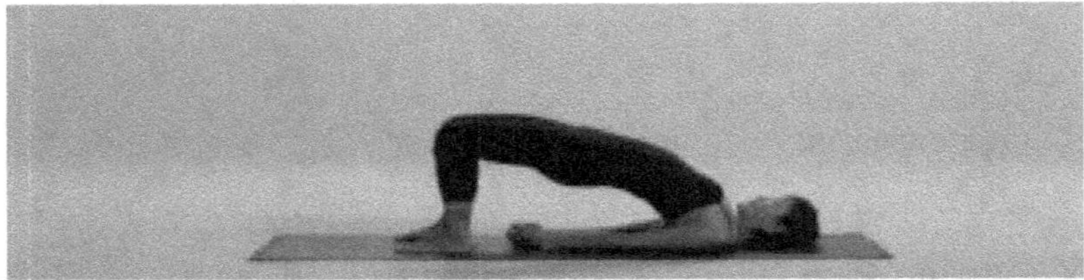

Figure 34

Corpse Pose

Like a life cycle, yoga poses end in this stage. It gives a moment of relaxation, but it is difficult for some people to stay still in this pose. The more you try this pose, the easier it gets into a relaxing, meditative stage.

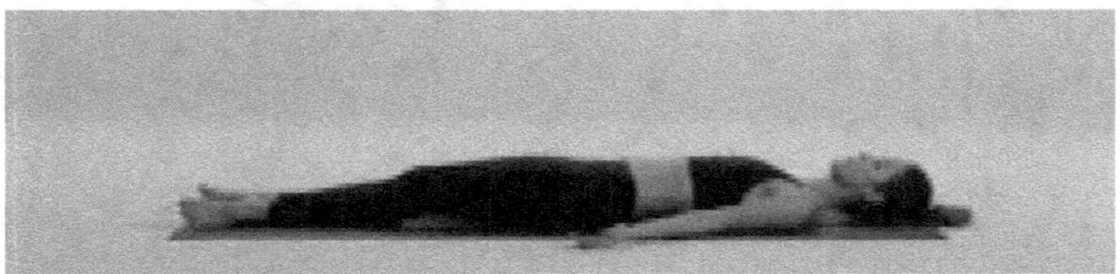

Figure 35

Meditation

Meditation is the practice that deals with focusing or clearing your thoughts with the use of combined physical and mental techniques.

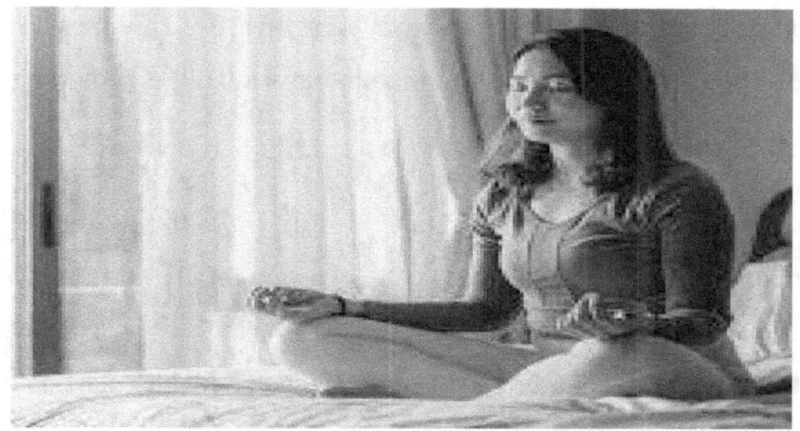

Figure 36

The reason why you should meditate is that it helps you to relax, lowers anxiety, lowers stress, lowers pain, and gives a better connection.

How to Meditate

1. To start meditation, look for a place where you can quietly and comfortably sit.
2. Then close your eyes and do nothing for a minute or thereabout.
3. Continue saying your mantra quietly inside for 4 minutes more. If thoughts interfere during this process, quickly return to saying your mantra inside quietly.

This instruction should only be followed for your first meditation.

Meditate every morning and every evening for 10-20 minutes. Make use of your mantra in your first meditation above. It is preferable to do your meditation before eating.

Quietly sit, close your eyes, and remain idle for a minute or thereabout. If you are interfered with by a thought, it is normal. After one or two minutes, in the same natural way that it came, and without moving your lips and tongue, quietly inside, start saying your mantra. Whenever you are interrupted by thoughts, quickly return to saying your mantra. When you are done meditating, lay down and observe a rest for 5-6 minutes.

Ideal Meditation Techniques for Beginners

Below are the various ideal meditation techniques for beginners to try:

- Breathing Meditations
- Mindfulness Meditations
- Focus Meditations
- Walking Meditations
- Progressive Muscle Relaxation Meditations
- Mantra Meditations

Breathing Meditations

- Breathe in for 6 seconds using your nose.
- Sustain your breath for 8 seconds.
- Exhale completely using your mouth, and purse the lips for 10 seconds.
- You can go through this breathing cycle over again up to 6 times.

This kind of breathing technique can shift your focus completely and your mind state.

Mindfulness Meditations

This meditation technique has to do with the ability to be present where you are.

- Remove your thoughts from the past or thoughts of the future.

- Engage in mindful breathing, guided imagery, or something like a fine picture from an art store meditation where you tune into your body.

- Give 100% of your attention to whatever you are doing at that moment.

- Take the time to breathe deeply or even scan through your body, working your way up from your toes to the top of your head.

Focus Meditations

This meditation is concerned with you looking at a particular object, like a candle or flower, with all mindfulness.

- Just select anything that stimulates your senses. For instance, if you have chosen a red rose, you could sit and look closely at the rose and imagine yourself touching it and feeling its velvety texture.

- You can begin as you choose an item of focus, such as a candle, and comfortably sit in front of it. As you breathe in and out, you will notice how the flame flickers or how the flame is made of several colors.

- Put your focus on the smells and the sounds, and experience what it is like to immerse yourself in the candle.

Mindful Walking Meditations

- This act is a practice whereby practitioners walk around the room while holding their hands in Shashu: holding one's hand closed in a fist behind the back, and the other hand closed within the fist.
- The kinhin is announced by the ringing of a bell twice.
- Take a walk-in silence by observing everything that is happening around your environment. For instance, you could observe the leaves on the trees if you are outside, feel the warmth of the sun, or pay attention to the sound your feet make as they hit the pavement or surface.

Progressive Muscle Relaxation Meditations

This type of meditation is a very classic one, which deals with the loosening and tightening of different muscles up and down the body.

- First, squeeze and release the large muscles of the body, either starting at the top of the head or the bottom of the feet.
- Stretch out the muscles at the hands and foot and contract it back again. Repeat this process four times.

Mantra Meditations

- If you want to practice mantra meditations, sit quietly on the ground and Centre yourself as you repeat your mantra 108 times. You could also use a prayer mala or a bead.
- Repeat a particular sound, known as a mantra. You can chant the mantra aloud or silently repeat it.
- A mantra is repeated for a 40-day cycle, but certainly, it is not necessary for a beginner.

Importance of an Individualized Treatment Plan Tailored to Each Patient's Specific Needs:

Personalized treatment plans are a very crucial part of effective treatment. Each individual who struggles with chronic disease has a specific treatment need. To handle these needs effectively and to achieve long-term recovery, it is very important to create a personalized treatment plan tailored to each patient's specific needs.

One important aspect of an individualized treatment plan is that it takes into account an individual's unique circumstances and experiences. These circumstances and experiences may include such factors as your age, sex, lifestyle behavior, and an existing mental health condition. Taking these factors into consideration, those in charge of treatment can create a workable plan that is tailored to each individual's specific needs, and this will help identify and address the actual cause of your condition.

A personalized treatment plan ensures that each individual gets the appropriate level and type of care they really need. For example, in some individuals, what is required is a more intensive treatment, such as inpatient care. On the other hand, outpatient or community-based care would be the right treatment option.

With this plan, individuals will feel more invested and engaged in their recovery. If treatment is tailored to an individual's needs, they will be more likely to feel noticed, seen, heard, and understood by their healthcare providers. It fosters trust and helps create a sense of partnership between the healthcare provider and the individual involved, which is crucial for successful recovery.

Personalized treatment plans can also help in addressing any challenges that may be peculiar to each individual. For instance, an individual with a transportation challenge could be included in a telehealth plan or possibly listed for transportation assistance.

In addition, a personalized treatment plan can help individuals develop skills and strategies for coping that are tailored to their specific needs. For instance, an individual battling with social anxiety may overcome this challenge with the use of Therapy focused on developing social skills and reducing stress. In contrast, an individual who is battling with the issue of trauma may overcome it with trauma-focused Therapy.

Personalized treatment plans can also help individuals develop a sense of ownership over their recovery, which will push them to remain committed.

A personalized treatment plan can also help in ensuring that individuals receive the most effective treatment possible. Taking into consideration each specific need, healthcare providers can develop a plan that is most likely to help them achieve lasting recovery.

Chapter Seven: Future Horizon and Research Avenues

Neuropathy is a painful and potentially damaging disorder mostly common among people with diabetes and majorly affects people with obesity. The major cause of this condition is still not clearly known.

Ongoing Research in The Field of Peripheral Neuropathy

The Neuropathy Centre at Weill Cornell Medicine is a committed Centre for translational and clinical research, which is aimed at increasing our understanding of the root cause of peripheral neuropathy and developing better therapies for the treatment of peripheral neuropathies.

Inflammatory Neuropathy & Autoimmune

The main focus of the research at these centers has been to diagnose and treat inflammatory neuropathy and autoimmune. Dr. Latov's laboratory has discovered anti-MAG and GM1 antibodies in neuropathy and has also developed diagnostic tests for the detection of these antibodies in patients with neuropathy.

Ongoing research is on the development and potential use of therapeutic anti-macrophage receptor CD204 antibodies for the treatment of inflammatory and diabetic neuropathies in experimental animal models of these diseases.

Dr. Latov has also served in various international committees for therapeutic trials; he was also involved in an ICE trial that led to the FDA approving intravenous immunoglobulin (IVIG) for CIDP, was a founding board member, and medical and research director of the Neuropathy Association. He has written over 100 publications in peer-reviewed journals, books, and chapters.

Dr. Russel Chin recently discovered nerve conduction studies, which have been used traditionally in the diagnosis of CIDP and can also be well used to detect ongoing disease activity.

Neuropathies as a Result of Improper Nutrition

Dr. Chin has contributed majorly to ensuring we understand the neuropathies resulting from celiac disease, and we have recently reported during our findings that a huge number of patients with neuropathy have levels of elevated vitamin B6 or mercury, which both can be toxic to nerves. The toxicity of B6 occurs due to excessive amounts of vitamin supplements, and toxicity of mercury usually happens when there is excessive consumption of seafood containing high levels of mercury. The required level of B6 is 2mg per day, but some daily supplements contain as high as 60 – 90 mg of B6. This improper nutrition can be corrected by modification of diets. In some patients, there is more than one cause for neuropathy, hence the need for holistic testing.

Areas of Interest for Further Research

Neuropathies resulting from metabolic syndrome or diabetes.

Ehlers Danlos syndrome.

Stem cell therapy in diabetic polyneuropathy: our breakthrough and further achievements.

Neuropathic pain: overall view of the present and looking into the future of therapies.

Peripheral neuropathy in metachromatic leukodystrophy: Present situation and future breakthrough.

Whole genome sequencing for idiopathic small fiber neuropathy.

There is a better future in research. In as much as research is still ongoing in determining the cause and remedies for peripheral neuropathies, the hope is very high that the actual cause and cure will be found. Your cooperation will make it a lot easier.

Possible Breakthroughs in Treatment and Interventions

Someday, Alpha lipoic acid/thioctic acid, HCN2 channel blockers, AAK1 inhibitors, and GABAergic transplants could be used to relieve pain in people who have exhausted the treatment regimens available for peripheral neuropathy.

Current pharmacotherapy for peripheral neuropathy

Tropical: Lidocaine and capsaicin are tropical agents that come with little risk of side effects. However, you are advised to use them peripherally or in the affected area, and they should be frequently applied.

Anticonvulsants: gabapentin and pregabalin are typical examples of anticonvulsants; they are used to relieve pain by modulating the hyperexcitable state of injured neurons. Gabapentinoids are associated with limited side effects such as constipation, nausea, vomiting, and mental imbalance.

Opioids: the use of opioids for neuropathic pain is not properly understood. Different clinical trials have indicated positive results in pain relief in patients; however, the period the therapy would be needed is not clear, knowing truly that neuropathic pain could last for a lifetime.

Novel neuropathic pain treatment as an option

Oxidative Stress and Antioxidant Agents: Oxidative stress occurs when the production of reactive oxygen species exceeds the cell's ability to detoxify it. An antioxidant agent such as alpha lipoic acid may provide a useful choice in treatment strategies for neuropathic pain due to their inhibitory effect on oxidative stress and ability to bring back that physiological redox balance. Currently, alpha lipoic acid and its dextrorotatory form, (+) – thioctic acid, are undergoing investigation for their effects on low back pain through oxidative stress relief to reduce damage to the nerve in sciatic pain.

Thioctic Acid in neuropathic pain management: Thioctic acid is a natural antioxidant that is available as a racemic (+/-) mixture. A recent study done in rats shows resolved analgesic sensitivity and reduced oxidative stress levels while applying thioctic acid.

Nucleotide 2 channel blockers

There are four categories of HCN ions: HCN1, HCN2, HCN3, and HCN4. HCN1 channels function mainly in the brain and heart;

HCN3 is more active in the central nervous system, while HCN2 and HCN4 channels are more active in the heart and central nervous system.

HCN2 Blockers: HCN2 blockers are currently being investigated for the treatment of neuropathic pain related to both inflammation and the hyper-excitability of ipsilateral spinal dorsal horn neurons.

Kinase 1 Inhibitors

Adapter Protein-2 Associated Kinase 1 Inhibitors: The adaptor-associated kinase 1 (AAK1) enzyme can be found predominately in the brain and the heart. The AAK1 enzyme was identified as having an impact on pain after investigators tested over 2,000 homozygous mouse knockout lines in acute and persistent pain behavior models. Meanwhile, the actual mechanism for the benefit of AAK1 inhibitors for neuropathic pain is unknown; it is believed to be related to alpha2 adrenergic signaling.

Evidence for AAK1 in Men and Mice: The study found that mice with the AAK1 knockout gene had markedly reduced responses to persistent pain. Researchers now induce persistent neuropathic pain through a different mechanism, ligating the L4 and L5 spinal nerves and resulting in immunity to mechanical allodynia. With these efforts, the creation of multiple oral compounds was successful. One of the compounds discovered, LP-935509, was associated with a dose-dependent impact on the reduction of pain behavior when studied in mice. Investigators found that higher doses of LP-935509 were found to have a similar effect on pain behavior compared to high-dose gabapentin. While LP-935509 is limited to mice study, there is another compound discovered during screening, BMS-986176, renamed LX9211, which is under investigation and has published results from two phases 1, randomized, double-masked, placebo-controlled studies. The main objective of both studies was to investigate the tolerability of LX9211 in healthy individuals. Therefore, it is expected that AAK1 inhibitors will make an entry into the market in the future as a better treatment option for neuropathic pain, even if it is used off-label.

Gabaergic Transplant

Gabaergic Transplant: Damage to the nervous system leading to interruption of this inhibitory pathway results in neuropathic pain.

Evidence for gabaergic Transplant: To investigate any benefit of MGE cell transplant, one study induced neuropathic pain in mice through transection of two of the three branches of the sciatic nerve.

Advancements in the Management of Peripheral Neuropathy

A common complication of diabetes is diabetes peripheral neuropathy; this condition affects approximately 50% of patients with diabetes. The complications associated with diabetes peripheral neuropathy are foot ulcers, chronic pain, and amputations, greatly affecting the patient's quality of life.

There is serious research going on to identify the real cure for all kinds of peripheral neuropathy, including diabetes peripheral neuropathy. Below, I shall discuss some recent advancements in the treatment of peripheral neuropathy.

Neuromodulation Technology: such as spinal cord stimulation, this has been approved by the United States Food and Drugs Administration (FDA) for managing painful diabetic neuropathy.

DF2755A: This substance has shown high potency in preventing and reversing peripheral neuropathy linked to non-ulcerative intestinal cystitis/bladder pain syndrome by directly inhibiting chemokine-induced excitation of sensory neurons.

Capsaicin Patch: Capsaicin 8% patch (Qutenza) is a treatment that is licensed in the EU/UK for neuropathic pain and has shown to be safe and effective for pain relief in patients suffering from chemotherapy-induced peripheral Neuropathy (CIPN).

ER Stress: Endoplasmic reticulum (ER) stress has also been implicated as a novel mechanism in the onset and progression of Diabetes Peripheral Neuropathy.

Mesenchymal stem cells (MSCs): mesenchymal stem cells have shown potential in treating neuropathy due to their ability to secrete a range of cytoprotective and anti-inflammatory factors.

We know there is still more to be done to understand the complex nature of peripheral neuropathy and develop effective treatments. Still, recent advancements in research have identified different promising therapeutic targets and interventions.

More research and clinical trials are necessary to authenticate these findings and to develop new therapies for neuropathy pains.

Chapter Eight: Inspiring Success Stories

Every patient suffering from peripheral neuropathy has a peculiar story to tell. I shall be sharing some stories of those who have successfully managed peripheral neuropathy, including myself, and are living a normal life presently.

Irene

Irene suffered multiple injuries to her knee, making her unable to walk as much as she desired. It was a very difficult task performing daily activities, including the ability to mow her lawn. After her first platelet-rich plasma injection at Carolina Pain Relief Centre, she felt so good she was now able to get out and cut the grass on her own! She is looking forward to her cell injection.

Roger

I love dancing, and over the past years, I developed peripheral neuropathy. I started losing the feeling in my feet, suffering from increased nerve pain, and having trouble picking things up. This condition was beginning to make getting around a lot more difficult. After my third platelet-rich plasma treatment at Carolina Pain Relief Centre, I was able to return to the things I loved without hindrances, and I'm ready for my trip to Portugal, where I will not have hindrances in any of those activities.

Keith

Keith had always lived a very active lifestyle but had to give up a lot of things he loved, such as basketball. After suffering from meniscus damage, he had arthroscopic surgery to remove the damaged piece nearly 20 years ago. Keith felt better at the time but slowly began to get worse, and he lost stability in his knee. He had to alter the way he walked, and he could only take one stair at a time.

If anyone were to bump into his knee, it would cause excruciating pain. After receiving Platelet Rich Plasma at

Carolina Pain Relief Centre, Keith is able to take the stairs again with no pain and has increased stability in his knee.

Jackie

Jackie is a musician who loves to play the fiddle and spend time with friends. She first came to us because she was suffering from

peripheral neuropathy, causing her foot and ankle pain and numbness as well as pain and weakness in her right hand, leaving her unable to do many of the things she loves. She even had to miss Thanksgiving dinner with her friends because her balance was so bad she was afraid to leave the house. She has been treated at

Carolina Pain Relief Centre with platelet-rich plasma, oxygen, and detox therapies.

She now has more feeling and balance and less pain in her feet and hands, and she has been able to lose weight.

Mary

Mary came to Carolina Pain Relief Centre seeking help for her peripheral neuropathy. She was unable to feel her feet. They felt like they were burning and cold at the same time and had electrical, shocking pains. After her first treatment, most of her pain was gone. After the second, her feet were no longer numb. She is now happy to say she has no more pain and no more numbness in her feet. Now that she can feel her feet, her balance is beginning to get better as a side effect.

Various Strategies and Positive Outcomes

The patients mentioned earlier have adopted natural treatment strategies to help them recover from peripheral neuropathy. In many cases, natural remedies have played an important role in preventing further nerve damage.

See below six natural remedies to help you overcome peripheral neuropathy.

Exercise: With exercise, many health challenges that lead to neuropathy are averted. For instance, diabetes can cause peripheral neuropathy. Exercise trims down blood sugar levels, which in turn reduces diabetes risk and other complications.

Change in diet: The leading cause of peripheral neuropathy is diabetes. It is good to go for diets that lower your blood sugar levels and ease your symptoms of neuropathy or prevent it entirely.

A diet low in simple carbohydrates and rich in fiber can help prevent the rise in blood sugar.

Quitting Smoking: One of the risk factors of peripheral neuropathy is smoking; this is because it narrows and damages peripheral blood vessels.

Avoiding smoking can improve blood flow around the body and make the blood vessels healthier.

Vitamins: Regular intake of vitamins and supplements has helped to improve nerve health and reduce symptoms of peripheral neuropathy.

Relaxation: Relax and take a deep breath; meditate; it will help relieve your pains.

Yoga, tai chi, and blended stretching have helped minimize stress and improve posture.

Use of alternative medicine: Try alternative medicine if you are suffering from peripheral neuropathy; combine acupuncture, chiropractic techniques, and energy-based modalities, such as Reiki.

To get the most out of alternative medicine, try combining your try with traditional treatments, such as exercise and medication.

Conclusion

This book, "Understanding and Managing Peripheral Neuropathy," has come at the right time as there are many who are suffering from peripheral neuropathy, with over 50% of the sufferers being diabetic patients.

Nephropathy affects the nerves outside the central nervous system that control muscle movement (motor nerves) and those that control sensations such as coldness or pain (sensory nerves). In most cases, internal organs, such as the bladder, blood vessels, heart, or intestines, are also affected.

Peripheral Nephropathy comes in three different forms, namely motor neuropathy, sensory neuropathy, and diabetic neuropathy.

More than half of those with diabetes also develop neuropathy.

Peripheral neuropathy can be diagnosed using these methods: blood tests, x-ray examination, nerve function tests, nerve biopsy, and skin biopsy. There are five ways to take charge of your emotions and cultivate better thoughts. – practice self-care, - manage your stress level, - talk about how you are feeling, - control those feelings you can, - seek physical relief from pain.

To enable you to cope with peripheral neuropathy, you need to set your priorities right, accept and acknowledge your condition, and always visit your therapist.

The comprehensive plans to relieve your pains are to ensure prevention, early diagnosis, and prompt treatment, deal with other health challenges, maintain a reduced weight all the time, eat a good diet, go for fruits, engage in regular exercise, and always manage your stress.

The following medications are very good pain relievers and symptom managers: Tricyclic antidepressants (TCAs) and Serotonin-noradrenaline reuptake inhibitors (SNRIs); Little opioids (Tramadol, tapentadol, morphine, and oxycodone; and None-steroidal anti-inflammatory drugs (diclofenac, and indomethacin).

There are a lot of physical therapies, as discussed in this book, but I focused on neurological physical therapy and occupational physical therapies. You can also consider alternative treatments such as acupuncture, chiropractic, reiki, and yoga.

Dr. Latov has discovered anti-MAG and GM1 antibodies in neuropathy and also developed diagnostic tests for detecting these antibodies in patients with neuropathy. Research is still ongoing to create and use therapeutic anti-macrophage receptors CD204 antibodies for the treatment of inflammatory and diabetic neuropathies.

There are a lot of success stories from those who have successfully managed their peripheral neuropathy.

Conclusively, you will have to follow the steps I highlighted in this book in order to experience positive outcomes in your condition and pains; there should be changes in lifestyle: exercise, modification in diet, quitting, vitamins, good relaxation, and lastly, use of alternative medicine.

Appendix

Resources and References

WEBSITES:

1. WebMD: Www.webmd.com

2. Healthline: Www.healthline.com

3. Institute for Advanced Reconstruction:
   Www.advancedreconstruction.com

4. Fidel Integrated Medical Solutions: Www.fidelintegrated.com

5. Myoclonic Labs: Www.news.myocliniclabs.com

Research Papers On Peripheral Neuropathy

1. DIAGNOSIS OF PERIPHERAL NEUROPATHY by HC Lehman

2. JOURNAL OF PERIPHERAL NERVOUS SYSTEM by Giuseppe Lauria, MD.

3. PERIPHERAL NEUROPATHY by Dr. Melissa Gouveia

4. PERIPHERAL NEUROPATHY by John D England, MD; Arthur K Asbury, MD.

5. WHAT IS PERIPHERAL NEUROPATHY? By Dr. Helen Webberley, MBChB, MRCGP, MFSRH

SUPPORT GROUPS FOR PERIPHERAL NEUROPATHY

1. FOUNDATION FOR PERIPHERAL NEUROPATHY

2. GUILLAIN BARRE SYNDROME SUPPORT GROUP

3. CHARCOT-MARIA-TOOTH UK

4. DIABETIC NEUROPATHY SUPPORT GROUP

5. WESTERN NEUROPATHY ASSOCIATION

6. NEUROPATHY ACTION FOUNDATION

INDEX

www.ingramcontent.com/pod-product-compliance
Lightning Source LLC
Chambersburg PA
CBHW071042250726
48653CB00005B/1953